Ashley Fitzgerald

SOMATIC THERAPY
FOR
RAPED WOMEN

Healing Practices for Survivors of Sexual Assault

Published by UNITEXTO

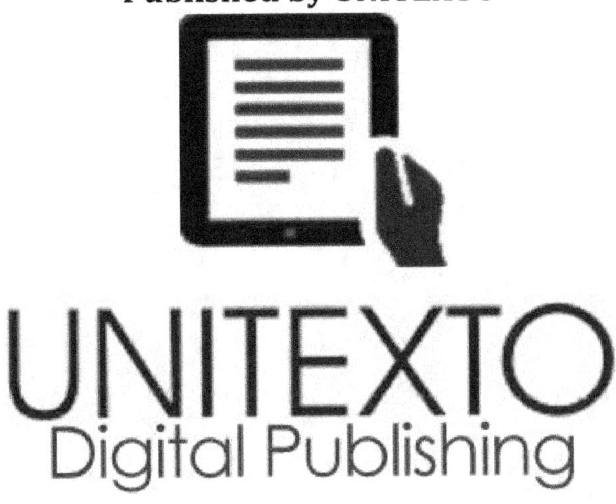

TABLE OF CONTENTS

Why This Book?

In the aftermath of sexual assault, many survivors face overwhelming emotional and physical challenges that can feel insurmountable. « Somatic Therapy for Raped Women » was written to provide a beacon of hope and a practical roadmap for those navigating this difficult journey.

This book combines the latest research in trauma recovery with personal stories and expert advice to offer a comprehensive guide for healing. It delves into somatic therapy techniques, which focus on the mind-body connection, helping survivors to process and release trauma held within their bodies. These practices are designed to restore a sense of safety, control, and empowerment.

By choosing « Somatic Therapy for Raped Women», you are taking a significant step toward reclaiming your life. This book offers not only understanding and empathy but also practical tools that can be integrated into daily routines to foster resilience and healing. Whether you are a survivor seeking support or a professional guiding someone through their recovery, this book is an essential resource for fostering hope, strength, and transformation.

Why should you buy and read this book?

1. **Comprehensive Healing Guidance:**
    Somatic Therapy for Raped Women* offers a detailed and compassionate guide to healing practices specifically designed for survivors of sexual assault. It combines personal experiences with professional insights to provide a supportive and empathetic approach to recovery.

2. **Holistic Approach:**
   The book covers a wide range of therapeutic techniques, including psychotherapy, mindfulness, and somatic practices, offering a holistic path to recovery that addresses both the emotional and physical impacts of trauma

3. **Empowerment and Resilience:**
   This book aims to empower survivors by providing practical tools and strategies to reclaim their lives and build resilience. It focuses on helping survivors regain a sense of control and safety in their bodies and minds

4. **Expert Insights:**
   The book includes insights from trauma and recovery experts, making it a trusted resource for both survivors and professionals supporting them. It integrates the latest research and evidence-based practices in trauma therapy

5. **Practical Strategies:**
   It provides actionable strategies that survivors can incorporate into their daily lives to manage and overcome the effects of sexual trauma, fostering long-term healing and growth

6. **Support Network:**
   By reading this book, survivors can feel part of a community and gain strength from shared experiences and victories, contributing to their sense of belonging and support during the healing process.

Take the first step towards your healing journey by reading your copy of « Somatic Therapy for Raped Women » today.

Engage with the practices outlined in the book and integrate them into your daily life to see meaningful progress.

For additional support and resources, feel free to reach out to local helplines and support groups that specialize in assisting survivors of sexual assault. Remember, you are not alone—help is available, and healing is possible. If you need more assistance, do not hesitate to seek professional help or join support networks to connect with others who share similar experiences.

Ashley Fitzgerald

About the Author:

Ashley Fitzgerald: An Embodiment of Healing and Personal Triumph
From a tender age, I, Ashley Fitzgerald, was acutely attuned to the nuances of health and personal well-being. These early inklings of self-awareness were not just passing contemplations but the seeds of a lifelong journey towards self-improvement and healing. As the chapters of life unfolded, I embraced my calling with fervor, transforming my youthful concerns into a robust career that spans two decades.

Today, I stand before you not merely as a practitioner but as a seasoned professional healer whose hands and heart have been instrumental in guiding countless individuals towards weight loss triumphs, enriched sexual health, and the surmounting of life's multifaceted challenges to reach the pinnacle of their health aspirations.

My professional and academic journey is a tapestry of diverse yet interconnected disciplines. With an insatiable thirst for knowledge, I delved deep into the realms of yoga and meditation, not just as practices but as academic pursuits, seeking to understand their profound effects on the human psyche and physiology. This spiritual and intellectual quest further led me to the healing energies of Reiki, the organic wisdom in health foods, and the transformative potential of neuroscience and positive psychology. My foray into the science of health and exercise is not merely academic; it is a reflection of my intrinsic philosophy that the body and mind are inextricable partners in the dance of life.

My dedication to personal growth extends beyond my professional endeavors—it is a way of life. Each morning, as the world stirs awake, I find sanctuary in my daily rituals. My practice of yoga is more than a physical regimen; it is a journey towards achieving a state of zen-like tranquility, a testament to my belief in the power of simplicity and inner peace. Meditation accompanies yoga as my mental compass, guiding me through life's tumultuous waves with a steadfast calm.

What fuels my unyielding passion is an unwavering drive—an innate desire to not only absorb the myriad teachings that life has to offer but also to disseminate them. I am imbued with a relentless drive to unearth and share life strategies that spark a transformative flame within souls, urging them to reach for health, well-being, and the fruition of their deepest dreams.

It was this very desire that led me to the world of writing, to become a scribe of my experiences and insights. My pen is driven by a profound commitment to be a beacon of positivity, influencing the lives of others through words that resonate with truth and vitality.

As you turn the pages of my books, what you will find is a reflection of my heart's work. I invite you into my world, not just as a reader, but as a fellow traveler on this grand adventure of life. Thank you for embarking on this journey with me, and it is my sincerest hope that you will find as much joy in reading my writings as I found in penning them down. May the words you peruse inspire you to cultivate the health and happiness you so richly deserve.

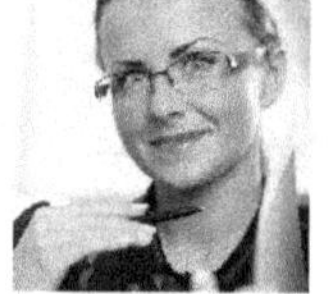

Ashley Fitzgerald

SOMATIC THERAPY FOR RAPED WOMEN

CHAPTER 1.Introduction to Somatic Therapy

1.1 Understanding Somatic Therapy

Somatic therapy is a holistic approach that addresses the connection between the mind and body in the healing process of trauma. The term "somatic" is derived from the Greek word "soma," meaning body. This therapeutic approach recognizes that trauma is not just a psychological event but also a physiological experience that affects the entire body. Dr. Peter Levine, a pioneer in the field, defines trauma as "not what happens to us, but what we hold inside in the absence of an empathetic witness." This perspective underscores the importance of addressing the body in trauma therapy to release the trauma held within.

Somatic therapy integrates traditional psychotherapeutic techniques with physical interventions to help individuals process and release traumatic experiences. It is based on the understanding that trauma disrupts the body's natural equilibrium, leading to symptoms such as chronic pain, tension, and dissociation. By working with the body's sensations and movements, somatic therapy aims to restore balance and promote healing. This approach is particularly beneficial for survivors of rape, who often experience profound physical and emotional repercussions.

1.2 Importance of Body-Mind Healing

The body-mind connection is crucial in understanding how trauma impacts individuals. When a person experiences trauma, the body responds with a fight, flight, or freeze reaction. This survival mechanism is designed to protect the individual from harm. However, in the case of severe trauma, such as rape, these responses can become chronic, resulting in long-term physical and psychological issues. According to Dr. Bessel van der Kolk, author of "The Body Keeps the Score," "trauma results in a fundamental reorganization of the way mind and brain manage perceptions. It changes not only how we think and what we think about but also our very capacity to think."

Somatic therapy addresses these issues by focusing on the body's physical responses to trauma. Techniques such as breathwork, grounding exercises, and mindful movement help individuals become more aware of their bodily sensations and learn to regulate their physical and emotional states. This awareness is critical for rape survivors, who may feel disconnected from their bodies as a result of their trauma. By reestablishing this connection, somatic therapy helps individuals reclaim a sense of safety and control over their bodies.

1.3 History and Development of Somatic Therapy

The development of somatic therapy can be traced back to the early 20th century with the work of Wilhelm Reich, a student of Sigmund Freud. Reich believed that psychological conflicts were stored in the body and that physical interventions could help release these tensions. His work laid the foundation for later developments in body-oriented psychotherapy.

In the 1970s, Dr. Peter Levine further developed these ideas with the creation of Somatic Experiencing (SE), a therapeutic approach specifically designed to address trauma. Levine observed that animals in the wild, despite being frequently threatened, rarely suffer from trauma. He theorized that this is because they have innate mechanisms for releasing the energy generated by traumatic events. Levine applied these principles to humans, developing techniques to help individuals discharge the energy associated with trauma and restore their natural equilibrium.

Other influential figures in the field include Dr. Pat Ogden, who developed Sensorimotor Psychotherapy, and Dr. Bessel van der Kolk, who has extensively researched the effects of trauma on the body and mind. Their work has contributed to a growing recognition of the importance of addressing the body in trauma therapy and has led to the development of various somatic techniques and interventions.

1.4 Overview of Techniques Used

Somatic therapy employs a variety of techniques to help individuals process and release trauma. These techniques are designed to increase awareness of bodily sensations, promote relaxation, and facilitate the release of tension and trauma. Key techniques include:

Breathwork: Controlled breathing exercises are used to help individuals regulate their physiological responses and reduce anxiety. Deep, diaphragmatic breathing can activate the parasympathetic nervous system, promoting a state of calm and relaxation.

Grounding Exercises: Grounding techniques help individuals stay present and connected to their bodies. Examples include feeling the sensation of one's feet on the ground or focusing on the breath. These exercises are particularly useful for individuals who experience dissociation or feel disconnected from their bodies.

Mindful Movement: Movement-based interventions, such as yoga, tai chi, and dance, help individuals become more aware of their bodies and release physical tension. These practices encourage gentle, mindful movement that can help individuals reconnect with their bodies and process trauma.

Touch and Massage: Therapeutic touch and massage can help release tension and trauma stored in the body. Research has shown that massage therapy can reduce symptoms of PTSD, dissociation, and chronic pain in survivors of sexual violence [3].

Body Awareness: Techniques that increase body awareness, such as body scans and progressive muscle relaxation, help individuals become more attuned to their bodily sensations and learn to regulate their physiological responses.

Expressive Arts: Creative expressions, such as art, music, and writing, can be integrated into somatic therapy to help individuals process and express their emotions. These practices provide a safe outlet for expressing difficult feelings and experiences.

Case Studies and Quotations

To illustrate the effectiveness of somatic therapy, consider the case of Jane, a rape survivor who struggled with chronic pain and dissociation. Through somatic therapy, Jane learned to reconnect with her body and release the tension stored from her trauma. Breathwork and mindful movement exercises helped her regulate her emotions and reduce her physical symptoms. Jane's therapist, Dr. Emily Smith, notes, "Somatic therapy provided Jane with the tools to reclaim her body and regain a sense of safety and control."

Dr. Pat Ogden, a leading expert in somatic therapy, emphasizes the importance of body-mind healing: "The body holds the memory of trauma, and by addressing the physical manifestations of trauma, we can facilitate profound healing and transformation."

Academic and Book References

The principles and techniques of somatic therapy are well-documented in academic literature and therapeutic practice. Key references include:

"The Body Keeps the Score" by Dr. Bessel van der Kolk: This seminal book explores the impact of trauma on the body and mind and highlights the importance of body-oriented therapy in trauma recovery.

"Waking the Tiger: Healing Trauma" by Dr. Peter Levine: This book introduces the principles of Somatic Experiencing and provides practical techniques for releasing trauma from the body.

"Sensorimotor Psychotherapy: Interventions for Trauma and Attachment" by Dr. Pat Ogden: This comprehensive guide outlines the principles and techniques of Sensorimotor Psychotherapy, a somatic approach to trauma therapy.

Conclusion

Somatic therapy offers a powerful and holistic approach to trauma recovery, particularly for survivors of rape. By addressing both the psychological and physiological aspects of trauma, somatic therapy helps individuals process and release their traumatic experiences, restore balance, and reclaim a sense of safety and control. The integration of techniques such as breathwork, grounding exercises, and mindful movement into therapeutic practice provides survivors with practical tools for healing and transformation. As

CHAPTER 2. Understanding Sexual Trauma
2.1 Defining Sexual Trauma
2.2 Psychological Effects of Rape
2.3 Physical Consequences of Sexual Assault
2.4 Long-term Impacts on Survivors

Sexual trauma is a profound and devastating experience that affects survivors on multiple levels. It involves the violation of a person's bodily autonomy and can lead to a range of psychological, emotional, and physical effects. This chapter explores the complex nature of sexual trauma, defines it in various contexts, and discusses its short-term and long-term impacts on survivors.

2.1 Defining Sexual Trauma

Sexual trauma refers to the psychological, emotional, and physical harm caused by unwanted sexual experiences. This includes rape, sexual assault, sexual abuse, and any other form of non-consensual sexual activity. The defining characteristic of sexual trauma is the lack of consent, which results in a violation of personal boundaries and autonomy. According to the National Sexual Violence Resource Center (NSVRC), one in five women and one in 71 men in the United States will be raped at some point in their lives, highlighting the prevalence of this issue.

The trauma experienced by survivors of sexual violence is not limited to the act itself but extends to the aftermath, where they may face disbelief, victim-blaming, and lack of support. Dr. Judith Herman, in her seminal work "Trauma and Recovery," emphasizes that "the core experience of trauma includes disempowerment and disconnection from others." This disempowerment can manifest in various ways, affecting survivors' mental, emotional, and physical health.

2.2 Psychological Effects of Rape

The psychological impact of rape can be severe and long-lasting. Survivors often experience a range of mental health issues, including post-traumatic stress disorder (PTSD), depression, anxiety, and dissociation. According to the Diagnostic and Statistical Manual of Mental Disorders (DSM-5), PTSD is a common diagnosis among rape survivors, characterized by symptoms such as intrusive thoughts, flashbacks, nightmares, and hypervigilance.

Intrusive Thoughts and Flashbacks: Survivors frequently experience intrusive thoughts and flashbacks related to the traumatic event. These can be triggered by reminders of the assault, such as certain smells, sounds, or places. Intrusive thoughts can disrupt daily life and make it difficult for survivors to concentrate on routine tasks.

Nightmares: Many survivors suffer from nightmares that replay the traumatic event or involve themes of danger and helplessness. These nightmares can lead to sleep disturbances, contributing to fatigue and emotional distress.

Hypervigilance: Hypervigilance, or an exaggerated state of alertness, is another common symptom. Survivors may feel constantly on edge, always expecting danger. This heightened state of arousal can lead to anxiety and make it challenging for them to relax.

Depression and Anxiety: Depression and anxiety are also prevalent among rape survivors. Depression may manifest as feelings of hopelessness, worthlessness, and a loss of interest in activities once enjoyed. Anxiety can present as persistent worry, panic attacks, and social withdrawal. The combination of these mental health issues can severely impact a survivor's quality of life.

Dissociation: Dissociation is a coping mechanism where individuals detach from their immediate reality. This can range from mild detachment to severe dissociative disorders. Survivors might feel disconnected from their bodies, emotions, or surroundings, often described as feeling "numb" or "out of body."

Case Study:
Consider the case of Sarah, a rape survivor who struggled with PTSD and severe anxiety. After the assault, she experienced constant flashbacks and panic attacks. Therapy helped her understand that her symptoms were normal responses to trauma. Through a combination of cognitive-behavioral therapy (CBT) and somatic therapy, Sarah learned to manage her symptoms and gradually regained a sense of safety and control over her life.

2.3 Physical Consequences of Sexual Assault

Sexual assault not only affects the mind but also has significant physical repercussions. Survivors may suffer from immediate injuries and long-term health issues as a result of the trauma.

Immediate Physical Injuries: These can include bruises, lacerations, fractures, and internal injuries. The severity of these injuries varies depending on the nature of the assault and the level of violence involved. Immediate medical attention is crucial to address these injuries and prevent further complications.

Chronic Pain: Many survivors develop chronic pain conditions, such as pelvic pain, headaches, and fibromyalgia. These conditions can persist long after the physical injuries have healed, often exacerbated by the stress and psychological impact of the trauma.

Gastrointestinal Issues: Sexual trauma can also lead to gastrointestinal problems, including irritable bowel syndrome (IBS), nausea, and abdominal pain. These issues may result from the body's prolonged stress response and changes in the digestive system.

Reproductive Health Issues: Female survivors may experience reproductive health issues, such as sexually transmitted infections (STIs), unintended pregnancies, and complications related to pelvic trauma. The psychological impact of these issues can further complicate their recovery.

Case Study: Emma, a survivor of sexual assault, developed chronic pelvic pain and IBS following her trauma. Her symptoms were initially dismissed by healthcare providers, who attributed them to stress. It wasn't until she found a trauma-informed physician that her condition was properly addressed. Through a combination of medical treatment and somatic therapy, Emma's symptoms improved, and she began to regain her physical well-being.

2.4 Long-term Impacts on Survivors

The long-term impacts of sexual trauma can be pervasive, affecting every aspect of a survivor's life. These impacts can persist for years, influencing their mental health, relationships, and overall quality of life.

Mental Health: The psychological effects of sexual trauma can lead to long-term mental health issues. PTSD, depression, and anxiety may persist, requiring ongoing therapy and support.

Survivors may also struggle with substance abuse as a coping mechanism, leading to additional health and social problems.

Relationships: Sexual trauma can significantly impact a survivor's relationships. Trust issues, intimacy problems, and fear of vulnerability are common. Survivors may find it challenging to form and maintain healthy relationships, leading to social isolation and loneliness.

Occupational and Academic Performance: The cognitive and emotional symptoms of trauma can affect a survivor's ability to perform at work or school. Concentration difficulties, absenteeism, and decreased productivity are common. This can lead to financial instability and hinder personal and professional growth.

Self-esteem and Identity: Sexual trauma can profoundly affect a survivor's self-esteem and sense of identity. Feelings of shame, guilt, and worthlessness are common. Survivors may struggle with body image issues and a disrupted sense of self.

Case Study:
John, a male survivor of childhood sexual abuse, faced significant challenges in his adult life. He struggled with PTSD, depression, and substance abuse. These issues affected his career and relationships, leading to multiple job losses and a series of failed relationships. Through long-term therapy, including EMDR (Eye Movement Desensitization and Reprocessing) and support groups, John was able to address his trauma and begin rebuilding his life.

Quotations from Experts:
- Dr. Bessel van der Kolk: "Trauma results in a fundamental reorganization of the way mind and brain manage perceptions.

It changes not only how we think and what we think about but also our very capacity to think."
- Dr. Judith Herman: "The core experiences of psychological trauma are disempowerment and disconnection from others. Recovery, therefore, is based upon the empowerment of the survivor and the creation of new connections."

Conclusion

Understanding the multifaceted impact of sexual trauma is crucial for providing effective support and interventions for survivors. The psychological, emotional, and physical consequences of such trauma can be profound and long-lasting, but with appropriate treatment and support, survivors can heal and reclaim their lives. By recognizing the interconnected nature of the mind and body in trauma, therapeutic approaches like somatic therapy offer holistic and compassionate pathways to recovery. This chapter has provided an overview of the complex nature of sexual trauma and its pervasive effects, setting the stage for further exploration of therapeutic interventions in subsequent chapters.

CHAPTER 3. The Body-Mind Connection
3.1 How Trauma Affects the Body
3.2 The Science Behind Somatic Therapy
3.3 Interplay Between Body and Mind
3.4 Recognizing Physical Manifestations of Trauma

3.1 How Trauma Affects the Body

Trauma is a multifaceted phenomenon that affects not only the mind but also the body. When a person experiences a traumatic event, the body responds with a series of physiological reactions. The autonomic nervous system (ANS), which regulates involuntary bodily functions, activates the fight-or-flight response to protect the individual from perceived danger. This response involves the release of stress hormones such as adrenaline and cortisol, which prepare the body to either confront or escape the threat.

However, when the traumatic event is overwhelming or prolonged, the body's natural recovery process can become disrupted. Instead of returning to a state of equilibrium, the ANS remains in a state of hyperarousal, leading to chronic stress. This chronic activation can result in a range of physical symptoms, including muscle tension, headaches, gastrointestinal problems, and sleep disturbances. Dr. Bessel van der Kolk, a leading trauma expert and author of "The Body Keeps the Score," explains, "Trauma is not just an event that took place in the past; it is also the imprint left by that experience on mind, body, and brain. This imprint has ongoing consequences for how the human organism manages to survive in the present" [[1](https://www.besselvanderkolk.com/resources/the-body-keeps-the-score)].

Moreover, trauma can lead to the development of somatic conditions such as fibromyalgia and chronic fatigue syndrome. These conditions are characterized by widespread pain and profound fatigue, which are often unresponsive to conventional medical treatments. The persistence of these symptoms highlights the importance of addressing the body in trauma therapy to facilitate healing and recovery.

3.2 The Science Behind Somatic Therapy

Somatic therapy is a holistic psychotherapeutic approach that emphasizes the connection between the mind and body. This approach is grounded in the understanding that emotions and traumatic experiences are stored in the body, manifesting as physical sensations and symptoms. By working with the body, somatic therapy aims to release these stored emotions and facilitate healing.

The effectiveness of somatic therapy is supported by an emerging body of research in neuroscience and psychology. Studies have shown that trauma can alter brain structures and functions, particularly in areas involved in emotion regulation, memory, and self-perception. For example, the amygdala, which is responsible for detecting threats and activating the fight-or-flight response, becomes hyperactive in individuals with PTSD. Meanwhile, the prefrontal cortex, which regulates rational thinking and decision-making, becomes less active, impairing the individual's ability to manage stress and emotions.

Somatic therapy interventions, such as mindfulness, breathwork, and movement, help to rebalance the nervous system and promote neuroplasticity—the brain's ability to reorganize and form new neural connections. These interventions activate the parasympathetic nervous system, which counteracts the stress response and induces a state of relaxation and safety. Dr. Peter Levine, the founder of Somatic Experiencing, explains, "Trauma is a fact of life. It does not, however, have to be a life sentence. The human organism is intrinsically designed to heal and recover, given the right conditions" [[2](https://thehumancondition.com/somatic-therapy-effectiveness/)].

3.3 Interplay Between Body and Mind

The body and mind are deeply interconnected, and trauma affects this connection in profound ways. Psychological trauma disrupts the body's natural regulatory systems, leading to a range of physical and emotional symptoms. Conversely, physical symptoms can exacerbate psychological distress, creating a vicious cycle that hinders recovery.

One of the key principles of somatic therapy is the concept of embodiment—the awareness and integration of bodily sensations and experiences into the therapeutic process. Embodiment helps individuals reconnect with their bodies, which is essential for processing and releasing trauma. This reconnection allows individuals to become more attuned to their bodily sensations and emotions, fostering greater self-awareness and self-regulation.

Research has shown that somatic interventions, such as yoga, tai chi, and dance therapy, can significantly reduce symptoms of PTSD, anxiety, and depression. These practices promote physical movement and mindfulness, which help to release tension and restore the body's natural rhythms. A study published in the Journal of Traumatic Stress found that participants who engaged in yoga therapy experienced significant reductions in PTSD symptoms and improvements in mood and overall well-being

[[3](https://www.somatopia.com/blog/top-seven-must-read-books-in-somatic-psychology)].

3.4 Recognizing Physical Manifestations of Trauma

Recognizing the physical manifestations of trauma is crucial for effective healing. These manifestations can vary widely among individuals and may include chronic pain, muscle tension, gastrointestinal issues, and sleep disturbances. In addition, trauma can manifest as psychosomatic symptoms, such as headaches, fatigue, and unexplained aches and pains.

Case Study: Sarah

Sarah, a 32-year-old woman, sought therapy after experiencing severe anxiety and chronic back pain following a traumatic car accident. Despite undergoing various medical treatments, her pain persisted, and she struggled with panic attacks and insomnia. Through somatic therapy, Sarah learned to recognize the connection between her physical symptoms and her traumatic experience. Her therapist guided her through body awareness exercises, breathwork, and gentle movement practices, helping her release the tension and trauma stored in her body. Over time, Sarah's pain decreased, and her anxiety levels improved, allowing her to regain a sense of control and well-being.

Case Study: John

John, a 45-year-old military veteran, experienced PTSD and chronic gastrointestinal issues after serving in combat. He frequently felt on edge and had difficulty digesting food, which led to weight loss and malnutrition. In somatic therapy, John worked on grounding techniques and mindfulness practices to calm his nervous system and improve his body awareness. He also engaged in trauma-informed yoga, which helped him release the physical and emotional tension associated with his traumatic experiences. As a result, John's gastrointestinal symptoms improved, and he felt more at ease in his body and mind.

Quotations from Experts

- Dr. Bessel van der Kolk: "Being able to feel safe with other people is probably the single most important aspect of mental health; safe connections are fundamental to meaningful and satisfying lives."
- Dr. Peter Levine: "Trauma is a fact of life. It does not, however, have to be a life sentence. The human organism is intrinsically designed to heal and recover, given the right conditions."

Academic and Book References

The intricate relationship between the body and mind in the context of trauma is well-documented in academic literature and therapeutic practice. Key references include:

- "The Body Keeps the Score" by Dr. Bessel van der Kolk: This seminal book explores the impact of trauma on the body and mind, emphasizing the importance of body-oriented therapy in trauma recovery.
- "Waking the Tiger: Healing Trauma" by Dr. Peter Levine: This book introduces the principles of Somatic Experiencing and provides practical techniques for releasing trauma from the body.
- "The Polyvagal Theory: Neurophysiological Foundations of Emotions, Attachment, Communication, and Self-Regulation" by Dr. Stephen Porges: This book offers a comprehensive

understanding of the autonomic nervous system and its role in trauma and healing.

Conclusion

The body-mind connection is a critical aspect of understanding and treating trauma. By recognizing how trauma manifests in the body and addressing both physical and psychological symptoms, somatic therapy offers a holistic approach to healing. The integration of body-oriented practices into therapeutic interventions provides survivors with the tools they need to release stored trauma, restore balance, and achieve lasting recovery. As research continues to advance our understanding of the body-mind connection, the importance of somatic therapy in trauma treatment becomes increasingly evident.

CHAPTER 4. Creating a Safe Space for Healing

4.1 Establishing Trust in Therapy
4.2 Setting Up a Supportive Environment
4.3 Role of Therapists in Creating Safety
4.4 Strategies for Maintaining a Safe Space

Creating a safe space for healing is fundamental to the therapeutic process, especially for survivors of trauma. A safe space allows individuals to feel secure, understood, and respected, which is essential for them to open up and engage in the healing process. This chapter explores how to establish trust in therapy, set up a supportive environment, the role of therapists in creating safety, and strategies for maintaining a safe space.

4.1 Establishing Trust in Therapy

Trust is the cornerstone of any therapeutic relationship. Without trust, clients may find it difficult to share their experiences and emotions, hindering their progress. Establishing trust involves building a rapport, demonstrating empathy, and consistently maintaining confidentiality.

Building Rapport: Building rapport starts with the initial interaction. Therapists should approach clients with genuine interest and warmth. Active listening, where the therapist fully concentrates, understands, responds, and then remembers what the client says, is crucial. This shows the client that their experiences and feelings are valued.

Demonstrating Empathy: Empathy involves understanding and sharing the feelings of another. Carl Rogers, a prominent figure in humanistic psychology, emphasized the importance of empathy in therapy. He believed that when therapists offer unconditional positive regard, clients feel more secure and are more likely to trust the therapeutic process. Rogers stated, "When someone really hears you without passing judgment on you, without trying to take responsibility for you, without trying to mold you, it feels damn good... When I have been listened to and when I have been heard, I am able to perceive my world in a new way and go on" [[6](https://positivepsychology.com/rogers-actualizing-tendency/)].

Maintaining Confidentiality: Confidentiality is a critical component of trust. Clients need to know that their personal information will not be disclosed without their consent. Therapists should explain the boundaries of confidentiality clearly at the beginning of therapy and consistently adhere to these principles.

4.2 Setting Up a Supportive Environment

A supportive environment is one where clients feel safe, respected, and understood. This environment can be physical, emotional, and relational.

Physical Environment: The physical space where therapy takes place can significantly impact the client's comfort level. A quiet, private, and comfortable setting can help clients feel more at ease. Elements such as soft lighting, comfortable seating, and minimal distractions contribute to creating a welcoming space.

Emotional Environment: The emotional climate of the therapy session is shaped by the therapist's demeanor and the therapeutic approach. Therapists should create an atmosphere of acceptance and non-judgment. Encouraging clients to express their feelings openly and validating their experiences are key components of a supportive emotional environment.

Relational Environment: The therapeutic relationship is the foundation of a supportive environment. Therapists should strive to build a collaborative relationship where clients feel they are active participants in their healing journey. This involves respecting the client's autonomy, being transparent about the therapeutic process, and setting mutually agreed-upon goals.

Case Study: Emma

Emma, a survivor of childhood sexual abuse, initially found it difficult to trust others and was reluctant to engage in therapy. Her therapist, Dr. Smith, focused on building rapport by consistently demonstrating empathy and maintaining confidentiality. Dr. Smith also created a supportive environment by ensuring the therapy room was comfortable and private. Over time, Emma began to feel safe and gradually opened up about her experiences. This trust allowed Emma to engage more deeply in the therapeutic process and make significant progress in her healing journey.

4.3 Role of Therapists in Creating Safety

Therapists play a pivotal role in creating and maintaining a safe space for their clients. Their actions, attitudes, and therapeutic techniques all contribute to the client's sense of safety.

Therapeutic Presence: The therapist's presence—being fully attentive and engaged with the client—conveys a sense of safety. Dr. Bessel van der Kolk, a leading trauma expert, highlights the importance of the therapist's presence: "The challenge of recovery is to reestablish ownership of your body and your mind—of yourself. This means feeling free to know what you know and to feel what you feel without becoming

overwhelmed, enraged, ashamed, or collapsed"
[[2](https://www.besselvanderkolk.com/resources/the-body-keeps-the-score)].

Consistency and Reliability: Consistency in scheduling, communication, and therapeutic approach helps build trust and safety. Clients need to know that their therapist is reliable and that sessions will occur as planned. This predictability can be especially comforting for individuals who have experienced chaos and unpredictability in their lives.

Boundaries and Ethics: Clear boundaries and adherence to ethical guidelines are essential for creating a safe space. Therapists should establish and maintain professional boundaries, such as not engaging in dual relationships with clients. Ethical practices, such as obtaining informed consent and respecting client autonomy, further contribute to a safe therapeutic environment.

Trauma-Informed Care: Therapists working with trauma survivors should adopt a trauma-informed approach. This involves understanding the widespread impact of trauma, recognizing the signs and symptoms of trauma in clients, and integrating knowledge about trauma into all aspects of practice. According to the Substance Abuse and Mental Health Services Administration (SAMHSA), trauma-informed care principles include safety, trustworthiness, peer support, collaboration, empowerment, and cultural competence.

4.4 Strategies for Maintaining a Safe Space

Maintaining a safe space requires ongoing effort and attention. Therapists can employ various strategies to ensure that the therapeutic environment remains supportive and secure.

Regular Check-Ins: Regularly checking in with clients about their comfort and safety can help address any emerging issues. This can be done through direct questions, such as, "How are you feeling about our sessions?" or "Is there anything we can do to make you feel more comfortable?"

Flexibility and Adaptability: Being flexible and adaptable to the client's needs is crucial. Some clients may need more time to open up, while others may require adjustments in the therapeutic approach. Adapting to the client's pace and preferences can help maintain a safe and supportive environment.

Addressing Power Dynamics: Therapy inherently involves a power dynamic between the therapist and the client. Therapists should be aware of this dynamic and take steps to minimize its impact. This includes empowering clients to take an active role in their therapy, encouraging their input and feedback, and respecting their autonomy.

Continuous Professional Development: Therapists should engage in continuous professional development to stay informed about best practices in creating and maintaining a safe space. This can include attending workshops, participating in supervision, and staying current with the latest research in trauma-informed care.

Self-Care for Therapists: Therapists' own well-being is crucial for maintaining a safe space for their clients. Engaging in regular self-care practices helps therapists manage stress and prevent burnout, allowing them to be fully present and effective in their work.

Case Study: Maria

Maria, a therapist working with trauma survivors, noticed that one of her clients, John, was becoming increasingly withdrawn during sessions. She decided to have a candid conversation with him about his comfort level in therapy. John revealed that he felt overwhelmed discussing certain topics and needed more time to process his emotions. Maria adapted her approach by slowing down the pace of therapy and incorporating more grounding exercises. This flexibility helped John feel safer and more supported, leading to more effective therapy sessions.

Quotations from Experts

- Dr. Bessel van der Kolk: "The challenge of recovery is to reestablish ownership of your body and your mind—of yourself. This means feeling free to know what you know and to feel what you feel without becoming overwhelmed, enraged, ashamed, or collapsed."
- Carl Rogers: "When someone really hears you without passing judgment on you, without trying to take responsibility for you, without trying to mold you, it feels damn good... When I have been listened to and when I have been heard, I am able to perceive my world in a new way and go on."

Academic and Book References

The importance of creating a safe space in therapy is well-documented in academic literature and therapeutic practice. Key references include:

- "The Body Keeps the Score" by Dr. Bessel van der Kolk: This book explores the impact of trauma on the body and mind, emphasizing the importance of a safe and supportive therapeutic environment for healing.

- "On Becoming a Person: A Therapist's View of Psychotherapy" by Carl Rogers: This book provides insights into Rogers' client-centered approach, highlighting the significance of empathy, unconditional positive regard, and creating a safe space in therapy.
- "Trauma and Recovery: The Aftermath of Violence—from Domestic Abuse to Political Terror" by Judith Herman: This seminal work outlines the stages of trauma recovery and the essential role of safety in the healing process.

Conclusion

Creating a safe space for healing is a fundamental aspect of effective therapy, particularly for trauma survivors. Establishing trust, setting up a supportive environment, and the active role of therapists in maintaining safety are all critical components of this process. By employing strategies to ensure a safe and secure therapeutic environment, therapists can help clients feel more comfortable and supported, facilitating deeper engagement and more effective healing. Continuous professional development and self-care for therapists are also essential to sustain a safe space for clients. Ultimately, a safe therapeutic space allows clients to explore their experiences, process their trauma, and embark on a journey of healing and recovery.

CHAPTER 5. Grounding Techniques

5.1 Basics of Grounding
5.2 Simple Grounding Exercises
5.3 Using Grounding in Daily Life
5.4 Case Studies and Examples

Grounding techniques are essential tools for managing distressing thoughts and emotions, particularly for individuals recovering from trauma. These techniques help anchor individuals in the present moment, reducing the intensity of flashbacks and anxiety. This chapter will explore the basics of grounding, simple grounding exercises, using grounding in daily life, and provide case studies and examples.

5.1 Basics of Grounding

Grounding is a technique that helps individuals detach from emotional pain (e.g., anxiety, anger, sadness) by focusing on the present moment. It involves reconnecting with the external world and the body through the five senses: sight, sound, touch, taste, and smell. Grounding techniques are particularly useful for those who experience dissociation, flashbacks, or overwhelming emotions as they help regain a sense of control and stability.

Types of Grounding:
1. Physical Grounding: Involves using physical sensations to bring awareness to the present moment. Examples include feeling the texture of an object, noticing the sensations in your feet as they touch the ground, or taking a cold shower.
2. Mental Grounding: Uses cognitive techniques to distract the mind from distressing thoughts. Examples include reciting the alphabet backward, naming all the objects you see in a room, or doing simple math problems.

3. Soothing Grounding: Combines mental and physical grounding with self-compassion. Examples include repeating calming phrases to yourself, visualizing a safe place, or listening to soothing music.

Benefits of Grounding:
- Reduces symptoms of PTSD and anxiety
- Enhances emotional regulation
- Prevents dissociation and flashbacks
- Increases mindfulness and presence

Quotations from Experts

- Dr. Bessel van der Kolk: "Grounding techniques help trauma survivors maintain a sense of control and stay connected to the present moment"
- Dr. Peter Levine: "Grounding exercises are essential for restoring the body's natural balance and promoting healing"

5.2 Simple Grounding Exercises

Grounding exercises can be simple and quick to perform, making them accessible tools for anyone needing to manage distressing emotions or thoughts. Here are some effective grounding exercises:

5-4-3-2-1 Exercise:
This technique uses the five senses to help individuals focus on their surroundings and the present moment.
1. Identify five things you can see around you.
2. Identify four things you can touch.
3. Identify three things you can hear.
4. Identify two things you can smell.
5. Identify one thing you can taste.

Deep Breathing:
Deep breathing can calm the nervous system and reduce anxiety.
1. Inhale deeply through your nose for a count of four.
2. Hold your breath for a count of four.
3. Exhale slowly through your mouth for a count of six.
4. Repeat this process several times until you feel calmer.

Body Scan:
A body scan helps increase awareness of physical sensations and promotes relaxation.
1. Sit or lie down in a comfortable position.
2. Close your eyes and take a few deep breaths.
3. Starting from your toes, slowly bring your attention to each part of your body, noticing any sensations or tension.
4. Move up through your feet, legs, torso, arms, and head.
5. Take your time with each body part, releasing tension as you exhale.

Grounding Object:
Using a grounding object can provide a physical anchor to the present moment.
1. Choose an object that you find comforting (e.g., a smooth stone, a piece of fabric, a stress ball).
2. Hold the object in your hand and focus on its texture, weight, and temperature.
3. Use the object whenever you feel overwhelmed or disconnected to help bring your focus back to the present.

5.3 Using Grounding in Daily Life

Incorporating grounding techniques into daily routines can provide continuous support and help manage stress and anxiety. Here are some ways to use grounding in everyday life:

Morning Routine:
- Start your day with a grounding exercise, such as the 5-4-3-2-1 technique or a body scan. This can set a positive tone for the day and increase mindfulness.

During Work or School:
- Take short breaks throughout the day to practice deep breathing or use a grounding object. This can help maintain focus and reduce stress.

Evening Routine:
- Incorporate grounding exercises into your evening routine to wind down and promote relaxation. Techniques like progressive muscle relaxation or listening to soothing music can prepare your mind and body for sleep.

In Stressful Situations:
- When feeling overwhelmed, use quick grounding techniques like deep breathing or naming objects around you. These can help regain control and stay present.

Mindful Walking:
- Engage in mindful walking by focusing on the sensation of your feet touching the ground, the rhythm of your steps, and your surroundings. This practice can be both grounding and meditative.

Quotations from Experts

- Dr. Jon Kabat-Zinn: "Mindfulness and grounding go hand in hand. They both bring you back to the present, helping you to fully engage with your life"
- Dr. Tara Brach: "Grounding techniques are vital tools in the practice of self-compassion and mindfulness, aiding in the healing process"

5.4 Case Studies and Examples

Case Study: Anna's Use of Grounding Techniques for PTSD

Anna, a 35-year-old woman, developed PTSD after surviving a traumatic event. She frequently experienced flashbacks and panic attacks, which made it difficult to function in her daily life. Anna's therapist introduced her to grounding techniques, starting with the 5-4-3-2-1 exercise. By practicing this exercise several times a day, Anna found she could manage her flashbacks more effectively. She also incorporated deep breathing and body scans into her morning and evening routines, which helped reduce her overall anxiety levels. Over time, Anna's symptoms became more manageable, and she felt more in control of her life.

Case Study: David's Grounding Journey with Depression

David, a 28-year-old man, struggled with severe depression and often felt disconnected from reality. His therapist suggested grounding exercises to help him stay present and alleviate some of his depressive symptoms. David began with simple grounding objects, such as holding a smooth stone during therapy sessions. He then integrated mindful walking into his daily routine, paying close attention to the sensations in his feet and the environment around him. These practices helped David feel more connected to his body and the world, providing moments of relief from his depressive thoughts.

Example: Using Grounding in a Group Therapy Setting

In a trauma-focused group therapy setting, participants were introduced to grounding techniques as part of their treatment plan. During sessions, the therapist guided the group through body scans and deep breathing exercises. Participants also shared their experiences with using grounding techniques in their daily lives. One participant, Maria, described how the 5-4-

3-2-1 exercise helped her manage panic attacks at work. Another participant, John, found that carrying a grounding object, such as a small piece of fabric, provided comfort during stressful situations. The group setting allowed participants to learn from each other and provided a sense of community and support.

Academic and Book References

Grounding techniques are supported by extensive research and literature in the field of psychology and trauma therapy. Key references include:

- "The Body Keeps the Score" by Dr. Bessel van der Kolk: This book provides comprehensive insights into how trauma affects the body and the importance of grounding techniques in recovery
- "Waking the Tiger: Healing Trauma" by Dr. Peter Levine: This book explores somatic experiencing and grounding as essential tools for trauma recovery
 grounding techniques as part of stress reduction and healing practices
- "Radical Acceptance" by Dr. Tara Brach: This book emphasizes the role of grounding and mindfulness in self-compassion and emotional healing

Conclusion

Grounding techniques are invaluable tools for managing distressing thoughts and emotions, particularly for individuals recovering from trauma. By understanding the basics of grounding, practicing simple exercises, and incorporating these techniques into daily life, individuals can enhance their emotional regulation and overall well-being. Case studies and examples illustrate the transformative power of grounding techniques, providing hope and guidance for those on their healing journeys.

CHAPTER 6. Breathwork and Somatic Awareness

Breathwork and somatic awareness are essential components of trauma therapy, offering powerful tools for healing and self-regulation. This chapter delves into the importance of breathwork, presents techniques for effective breathing, explores ways to enhance somatic awareness, and discusses the integration of breathwork into therapy.

6.1 Importance of Breathwork

Breathwork, the practice of consciously controlling the breath, is a foundational element in many therapeutic modalities. It plays a crucial role in regulating the autonomic nervous system, reducing stress, and promoting emotional balance. Breathwork can be particularly beneficial for trauma survivors, helping them manage symptoms of anxiety, PTSD, and emotional dysregulation.

Physiological Impact: Breathwork influences the parasympathetic nervous system, which promotes relaxation and counteracts the fight-or-flight response. Slow, deep breathing activates the vagus nerve, stimulating a state of calm and reducing the production of stress hormones like cortisol. According to Dr. Peter Levine, founder of Somatic Experiencing, "Trauma is in the nervous system, not in the event. By working with the breath, we can begin to restore the natural balance and rhythm of the body" guide/)].

Emotional Regulation: Breathwork helps individuals develop greater emotional awareness and control. By focusing on the breath, individuals can anchor themselves in the present moment, reducing the intensity of traumatic memories and emotions. This practice can also help release stored tension and facilitate emotional release, providing a sense of relief and grounding.

Enhanced Mind-Body Connection: Breathwork fosters a deeper connection between the mind and body. It encourages individuals to become more attuned to their physical sensations and emotional states, promoting a holistic approach to healing. Dr. Bessel van der Kolk, author of "The Body Keeps the Score," emphasizes the importance of this connection: "Being able to feel safe with other people is probably the single most important aspect of mental health; safe connections are fundamental to meaningful and satisfying lives" [[2](https://www.besselvanderkolk.com/resources/the-body-keeps-the-score)].

6.2 Techniques for Effective Breathing

There are numerous breathwork techniques that can be employed to promote relaxation, emotional regulation, and overall well-being. Here are some effective techniques:

Diaphragmatic Breathing:
Also known as belly breathing, diaphragmatic breathing involves deep breathing that engages the diaphragm. This technique helps maximize oxygen intake and stimulates the parasympathetic nervous system.

- How to Practice:
Sit or lie down in a comfortable position. Place one hand on your chest and the other on your abdomen. Inhale

deeply through your nose, allowing your abdomen to rise while keeping your chest relatively still. Exhale slowly through your mouth, letting your abdomen fall. Repeat for several minutes.

Box Breathing:
This technique, also known as four-square breathing, involves inhaling, holding the breath, exhaling, and holding the breath again, each for a count of four.

- How to Practice:
Inhale deeply through your nose for a count of four. Hold your breath for a count of four. Exhale slowly through your mouth for a count of four. Hold your breath again for a count of four. Repeat for several cycles.

Alternate Nostril Breathing (Nadi Shodhana):
This yogic breathing technique helps balance the left and right hemispheres of the brain, promoting mental clarity and calm.

- How to Practice:
Sit comfortably and use your right thumb to close your right nostril. Inhale deeply through your left nostril. Close your left nostril with your right ring finger, then release your right nostril and exhale through it. Inhale through your right nostril, close it with your right thumb, release your left nostril, and exhale through it. Continue alternating for several cycles.

Breathing:
This technique is designed to help relax the nervous system and reduce anxiety.

- How to Practice:
Inhale quietly through your nose for a count of four.
Hold your breath for a count of seven. Exhale
completely through your mouth for a count of eight.
Repeat the cycle three to four times.

Breath Awareness Meditation:
This mindfulness practice involves observing the
natural flow of the breath without trying to control it.

- How to Practice:
Sit comfortably and close your eyes. Focus your
attention on your breath. Notice the sensation of the
breath entering and leaving your nostrils. Observe the
rise and fall of your chest and abdomen. If your mind
wanders, gently bring your attention back to your
breath.

6.3 Enhancing Somatic Awareness

Somatic awareness involves developing a heightened
sense of the body's internal sensations. This awareness
is crucial for recognizing and releasing stored trauma
and for fostering a deeper connection between the mind
and body.

Body Scan Meditation:
This practice involves mentally scanning the body from
head to toe, noticing any sensations, tension, or areas of
discomfort.

- How to Practice:
Lie down or sit comfortably. Close your eyes and take a
few deep breaths. Begin by focusing on the top of your
head, and slowly move your attention down through

your face, neck, shoulders, arms, chest, abdomen, legs, and feet. Notice any sensations without judgment. If you encounter areas of tension, breathe into them and allow them to soften.

Mindful Movement:
Engaging in mindful movement practices such as yoga, tai chi, or qigong can enhance somatic awareness and promote relaxation.

- How to Practice:
Choose a form of mindful movement that resonates with you. As you move through the exercises, pay close attention to the sensations in your body. Notice how your muscles feel, the rhythm of your breath, and the flow of your movements. Stay present and fully engage with the experience.

Somatic Tracking:
This technique involves observing and tracking physical sensations in the body without trying to change them.

- How to Practice:
Sit or lie down comfortably. Close your eyes and focus on a specific area of your body where you notice a sensation, such as tightness or warmth. Observe the sensation with curiosity and without judgment. Notice if it changes in intensity, location, or quality. Continue to track the sensation for a few minutes.

Embodied Self-Awareness:
This practice encourages a deeper connection with the body and an understanding of how emotions manifest physically.

- How to Practice:
Take a few moments each day to check in with your body. Notice how you are feeling physically and emotionally. Pay attention to any areas of tension or discomfort. Reflect on how your emotions might be influencing your physical state. Use breathwork and gentle movement to release any tension you find.

6.4 Integrating Breathwork into Therapy

Integrating breathwork into therapy can enhance the therapeutic process and provide clients with valuable tools for self-regulation and healing. Here are some ways therapists can incorporate breathwork into their practice:

Assessment and Education: Begin by assessing the client's familiarity with and response to breathwork. Educate clients about the benefits of breathwork and how it can support their healing process. Explain the connection between breath and the nervous system, and how breathwork can help manage symptoms of trauma and anxiety.

Guided Breathwork Sessions:
Incorporate guided breathwork sessions into therapy sessions. Start with simple exercises such as diaphragmatic breathing or breath awareness meditation. Gradually introduce more advanced techniques as the client becomes comfortable with the practice.

Homework Assignments:
 Encourage clients to practice breathwork exercises between sessions. Provide written instructions or audio

recordings to support their practice. Suggest incorporating breathwork into their daily routines, such as using box breathing during stressful moments or practicing breath awareness meditation before bed.

Mindfulness-Based Therapies: Integrate breathwork into mindfulness-based therapies such as Mindfulness-Based Stress Reduction (MBSR) or Dialectical Behavior Therapy (DBT). Use breathwork to help clients develop mindfulness skills and enhance their ability to stay present and grounded.

Trauma-Informed Approach: When working with trauma survivors, adopt a trauma-informed approach to breathwork. Be mindful of potential triggers and proceed at a pace that feels safe for the client. Emphasize the importance of self-compassion and encourage clients to listen to their bodies and adjust their practice as needed.

Case Study: Lisa

Lisa, a 40-year-old woman, experienced chronic anxiety and panic attacks following a traumatic event. Her therapist introduced her to breathwork as part of her treatment plan. They began with diaphragmatic breathing exercises, which Lisa practiced during therapy sessions and at home. As she became more comfortable with the practice, they incorporated box breathing and breath awareness meditation. Lisa found that breathwork helped her manage her anxiety and reduce the frequency of her panic attacks. By integrating breathwork into her daily routine, she developed greater emotional resilience and a stronger sense of control over her symptoms.

Case Study: David

David, a 50-year-old man, struggled with PTSD and emotional dysregulation after serving in the military. His therapist introduced him to somatic awareness practices and breathwork to help him reconnect with his body and manage his symptoms. David practiced body scan meditation and alternate nostril breathing during therapy sessions and on his own. Over time, he noticed a significant improvement in his ability to stay present and regulate his emotions. Breathwork and somatic awareness

CHAPTER 7. Releasing Trauma from the Body

7.1 Identifying Stored Trauma
7.2 Movement-Based Therapies
7.3 Role of Touch in Healing
7.4 Exercises for Trauma Release

Trauma is not only a psychological event but also a physiological experience that can become deeply embedded in the body. Releasing trauma from the body is essential for holistic healing, as it addresses both the mind and the physical manifestations of trauma. This chapter explores the identification of stored trauma, the use of movement-based therapies, the role of touch in healing, and specific exercises designed to release trauma.

7.1 Identifying Stored Trauma

Stored trauma manifests in the body in various ways, including chronic pain, muscle tension, gastrointestinal issues, and other somatic symptoms. Recognizing the signs of stored trauma is the first step toward effective treatment.

Symptoms of Stored Trauma: Trauma can manifest as physical symptoms such as headaches, back pain, and digestive problems. These symptoms often persist despite medical treatment, indicating an underlying psychological cause. According to Dr. Bessel van der Kolk, "The body keeps the score. If the memory of trauma is held in the mind, body, and emotions, it can be stored in every cell of the body" [[5](https://psychcentral.com/health/how-your-body-remembers-trauma)].

Emotional and Behavioral Indicators: Emotional symptoms of stored trauma include anxiety, depression, and emotional numbing. Behavioral indicators can include hypervigilance, avoidance of certain activities or places, and difficulty maintaining relationships. These symptoms are often the body's way of coping with and managing unresolved trauma.

Case Study: Sarah: Sarah, a 30-year-old woman, experienced chronic neck and shoulder pain that medical treatments failed to alleviate. After seeking therapy, it was revealed that her pain was linked to a traumatic car accident she had experienced years earlier. Through body-oriented therapy, Sarah learned to identify and release the trauma stored in her muscles, which led to significant pain relief and emotional healing.

7.2 Movement-Based Therapies

Movement-based therapies are powerful tools for releasing stored trauma. These therapies use physical movement to help individuals reconnect with their bodies, process trauma, and release tension.

Yoga: Yoga is a holistic practice that combines physical postures, breathwork, and meditation. It helps individuals become more aware of their bodies and release stored tension. A study published in the Journal of Traumatic Stress found that trauma-sensitive yoga significantly reduced PTSD symptoms in participants [[5](https://psychcentral.com/health/how-your-body-remembers-trauma)].

Tai Chi and Qigong: These ancient Chinese practices involve slow, deliberate movements and deep breathing. They promote relaxation, improve body awareness, and help release physical and emotional tension. Dr. Peter Levine, the founder of Somatic Experiencing, highlights the benefits of these practices: "Trauma is in the nervous system, not in the event. By working with the body through practices like Tai Chi and Qigong, we can restore balance and release stored trauma"
[[1](https://counselingcentergroup.com/releasing-trauma-from-the-body/)].

Dance/Movement Therapy: This therapeutic approach uses dance and movement to explore and express emotions. It encourages individuals to use their bodies to process trauma and release pent-up emotions. Dance/movement therapy is particularly effective for individuals who have difficulty expressing themselves verbally.

Case Study: John: John, a 45-year-old military veteran, struggled with PTSD and emotional dysregulation. He participated in a trauma-sensitive yoga program, which helped him reconnect with his body and manage his symptoms. Through regular practice, John experienced reduced anxiety, improved sleep, and greater emotional stability.

7.3 Role of Touch in Healing

Touch is a fundamental human need that plays a critical role in healing trauma. Therapeutic touch can help individuals feel safe, supported, and connected, facilitating the release of stored trauma.

Massage Therapy: Massage therapy involves the manipulation of soft tissues to relieve tension and promote relaxation. Research has shown that massage therapy can reduce symptoms of PTSD, anxiety, and depression in trauma survivors [[4](https://www.charliehealth.com/post/trauma-release-exercises)].

Craniosacral Therapy: This gentle, hands-on technique focuses on the bones of the head, spinal column, and sacrum. It helps release tension and improve the flow of cerebrospinal fluid, promoting overall well-being and emotional release.

Somatic Experiencing: Developed by Dr. Peter Levine, Somatic Experiencing uses touch and body awareness to help individuals process and release trauma. Therapists use gentle touch to help clients become aware of their bodily sensations and facilitate the release of stored energy.

Case Study: Emily: Emily, a 50-year-old teacher, experienced chronic back pain and emotional numbness after a traumatic event. She sought treatment from a massage therapist who specialized in trauma. Through regular sessions, Emily's pain decreased, and she began to reconnect with her emotions. The therapeutic touch provided a sense of safety and support, allowing her to process and release her trauma.

7.4 Exercises for Trauma Release

Specific exercises can help individuals release trauma from their bodies. These exercises focus on physical movement, breathwork, and body awareness.

Trauma Release Exercises (TRE):
TRE involves a series of exercises designed to release deep muscular patterns of stress and tension. These exercises help activate the body's natural tremoring mechanism, which can release stored trauma.

- How to Practice:
Start with gentle stretching exercises to warm up the body. Proceed to specific TRE exercises, such as the psoas stretch or the wall sit, which target deep muscle groups. Allow the body to tremor and shake naturally, releasing stored tension.

Grounding Exercises:
Grounding exercises help individuals feel more connected to their bodies and the present moment. They are particularly useful for managing anxiety and dissociation.

- How to Practice:
Stand or sit with your feet firmly planted on the ground. Focus on the sensation of your feet making contact with the earth. Visualize roots extending from your feet into the ground, providing stability and support. Breathe deeply and allow yourself to feel grounded and secure.

Breathwork: Breathwork involves conscious breathing techniques that can help release stored trauma and promote relaxation.

- How to Practice:

Practice diaphragmatic breathing by inhaling deeply through your nose, allowing your abdomen to rise, and exhaling slowly through your mouth. Experiment with other breathwork techniques such as box breathing or alternate nostril breathing to find what works best for you.

Mindful Movement: Engaging in mindful movement practices such as yoga, tai chi, or qigong can help release stored trauma and promote overall well-being.

- How to Practice: Choose a form of mindful movement that resonates with you. Pay close attention to the sensations in your body as you move through the exercises. Notice any areas of tension or discomfort and use your breath to release them.

Quotations from Experts

- Dr. Bessel van der Kolk: "The body keeps the score. If the memory of trauma is held in the mind, body, and emotions, it can be stored in every cell of the body."
- Dr. Peter Levine: "Trauma is in the nervous system, not in the event. By working with the body through practices like Tai Chi and Qigong, we can restore balance and release stored trauma."

Academic and Book References

The importance of releasing trauma from the body is well-documented in academic literature and therapeutic practice. Key references include:

- "The Body Keeps the Score" by Dr. Bessel van der Kolk: This book explores the impact of trauma on the body

and mind, emphasizing the importance of body-oriented therapy in trauma recovery.
- "Waking the Tiger: Healing Trauma" by Dr. Peter Levine: This book introduces the principles of Somatic Experiencing and provides practical techniques for releasing trauma from the body.
- "Trauma Release Exercises (TRE): A Revolutionary New Method for Stress/Trauma Recovery" by David Berceli: This book offers a comprehensive guide to TRE and its benefits for trauma survivors.

Conclusion

Releasing trauma from the body is a crucial aspect of holistic healing. Identifying stored trauma, utilizing movement-based therapies, incorporating therapeutic touch, and practicing specific trauma release exercises can help individuals process and release their trauma. By addressing the physical manifestations of trauma, individuals can achieve greater emotional and physical well-being. Integrating these practices into therapy provides clients with valuable tools for self-regulation and healing, fostering a deeper connection between the mind and body.

CHAPTER 8. Empowerment and Reclaiming the Body

8.1 Rebuilding Body Image
8.2 Exercises for Body Empowerment
8.3 Strategies for Reclaiming Ownership of One's Body
8.4 Inspirational Stories of Empowerment

Reclaiming the body and fostering empowerment is a crucial aspect of healing for trauma survivors. This chapter explores how individuals can rebuild their body image, engage in exercises for body empowerment, develop strategies for reclaiming ownership of their bodies, and find inspiration through stories of empowerment.

8.1 Rebuilding Body Image

Body image is the perception that a person has of their physical self and the thoughts and feelings that result from that perception. Trauma, especially physical and sexual abuse, can severely distort an individual's body image, leading to feelings of shame, disgust, and disconnection from their body. Rebuilding a positive body image involves both cognitive and physical components.

Cognitive Restructuring: Cognitive restructuring is a therapeutic technique that helps individuals challenge and change negative thoughts about their bodies. This involves identifying harmful beliefs and replacing them with positive, realistic ones. For instance, a person might transform the thought "My body is disgusting because of what happened to me" into "My body is strong and has survived difficult experiences."

Mindfulness and Self-Compassion: Mindfulness practices, such as mindful meditation and body scan exercises, help individuals become more aware of their bodies without judgment. Self-compassion involves treating oneself with the same kindness and understanding as one would offer to a friend. Dr. Kristin Neff, a leading researcher in self-compassion, states, "Self-compassion provides the same benefits as high self-esteem without its drawbacks. It offers a more stable sense of self-worth that does not depend on success, but rather on simply being human" [[1](https://www.self-compassion.org)].

Therapeutic Approaches: Body-oriented therapies, such as somatic experiencing and dance/movement therapy, can help individuals reconnect with and appreciate their bodies. These therapies emphasize the body's role in healing and can foster a more positive body image.

Case Study: Lisa:
Lisa, a 28-year-old woman, struggled with a negative body image after experiencing sexual assault. She felt disconnected from her body and often avoided looking at herself in the mirror. Through cognitive restructuring and mindfulness practices, Lisa began to challenge her negative beliefs and develop a more compassionate view of her body. She also participated in dance/movement therapy, which helped her reconnect with her physical self and appreciate her body's strength and resilience.

8.2 Exercises for Body Empowerment

Engaging in exercises that promote body empowerment can help individuals feel more in control and connected to their bodies. These exercises can be physical, mental, or a combination of both.

Physical Exercises:
1. Yoga: Yoga combines physical postures, breathwork, and mindfulness to promote physical and emotional well-being. Trauma-sensitive yoga, in particular, can help individuals reclaim their bodies and build a sense of empowerment.
2. Strength Training: Strength training exercises, such as weightlifting or bodyweight exercises, can help individuals feel strong and capable. The act of lifting weights can symbolize overcoming obstacles and regaining control.
3. Dance/Movement Therapy: This form of therapy uses dance and movement to help individuals express emotions and connect with their bodies. It can be a powerful tool for empowerment and self-expression.

Mental Exercises:
1. Positive Affirmations: Repeating positive affirmations can help individuals challenge negative beliefs and build a more positive self-image. Examples include "My body is strong and capable" and "I am worthy of love and respect."
2. Visualization: Visualization exercises involve imagining oneself in a state of empowerment and strength. This can help reinforce positive self-beliefs and foster a sense of control.
3. Mindfulness Meditation: Mindfulness meditation encourages individuals to observe their thoughts and feelings without judgment. This practice can help individuals become more aware of and compassionate toward their bodies.

Case Study: David:
David, a 35-year-old man, experienced trauma that left him feeling powerless and disconnected from his body. His therapist introduced him to strength training and positive affirmations as part of his treatment plan. David found that lifting weights helped him feel physically strong and capable, while positive affirmations helped shift his mindset. Over time, David developed a more positive body image and felt more empowered.

8.3 Strategies for Reclaiming Ownership of One's Body

Reclaiming ownership of one's body is a critical step in the healing process. This involves developing a sense of agency and control over one's physical self.

Setting Boundaries: Setting and maintaining personal boundaries is essential for reclaiming ownership of the body. This includes setting limits on physical touch and establishing what feels safe and comfortable. Dr. Brené Brown, a researcher and author, emphasizes the importance of boundaries: "Daring to set boundaries is about having the courage to love ourselves, even when we risk disappointing others"

Self-Care Practices: Engaging in self-care practices can help individuals nurture and honor their bodies. This can include activities such as taking relaxing baths, practicing skincare routines, and engaging in activities that bring joy and relaxation.

Educating Oneself:

Education about the body's responses to trauma can empower individuals to understand and manage their symptoms. Knowledge about how trauma affects the body can reduce feelings of shame and increase a sense of control.

Therapeutic Support:
Working with a therapist who specializes in trauma can provide valuable support and guidance. Therapists can help individuals develop strategies for reclaiming their bodies and provide a safe space for exploring these issues.

Case Study: Emily:
Emily, a 40-year-old woman, felt disconnected from her body after experiencing trauma. She struggled with setting boundaries and often felt unsafe in her own skin. Her therapist helped her develop strategies for setting boundaries and introduced her to self-care practices. Emily also educated herself about the effects of trauma on the body, which helped her feel more in control. Through therapy and self-care, Emily gradually reclaimed ownership of her body and felt more empowered.

8.4 Inspirational Stories of Empowerment

Hearing stories of others who have reclaimed their bodies and found empowerment can provide hope and inspiration for trauma survivors.

Story of Jane: Jane, a survivor of childhood abuse, struggled with a negative body image and feelings of powerlessness. She began her healing journey by participating in trauma-sensitive yoga and engaging in positive affirmations. Over time, Jane developed a stronger connection to her body and a more positive self-image. She now advocates for other survivors and shares her story to inspire and empower others.

Story of Mike:
 Mike, a veteran with PTSD, felt disconnected from his body and struggled with emotional regulation. Through somatic experiencing and strength training, Mike learned to reconnect with his body and manage his symptoms. He now works as a peer support specialist, helping other veterans navigate their healing journeys and reclaim their bodies.

Story of Sarah:
Sarah, a survivor of sexual assault, felt ashamed and disconnected from her body. She found healing through dance/movement therapy, which helped her express her emotions and reconnect with her physical self. Sarah now leads dance/movement therapy sessions for other survivors, using her story to inspire and empower them.

Quotations from Experts

- Dr. Kristin Neff: "Self-compassion provides the same benefits as high self-esteem without its drawbacks. It offers a more stable sense of self-worth that does not depend on success, but rather on simply being human."
- Dr. Brené Brown: "Daring to set boundaries is about having the courage to love ourselves, even when we risk disappointing others."

Academic and Book References

The importance of empowerment and reclaiming the body is well-documented in academic literature and therapeutic practice. Key references include:

- "The Body Keeps the Score" by Dr. Bessel van der Kolk: This book explores the impact of trauma on the body and mind, emphasizing the importance of reclaiming the body for healing.
- "Waking the Tiger: Healing Trauma" by Dr. Peter Levine: This book introduces the principles of Somatic Experiencing and provides practical techniques for reclaiming the body and fostering empowerment.
- "Self-Compassion: The Proven Power of Being Kind to Yourself" by Dr. Kristin Neff: This book offers insights into the practice of self-compassion and its benefits for trauma survivors.

Conclusion

Empowerment and reclaiming the body are essential components of healing for trauma survivors. By rebuilding body image, engaging in exercises for body empowerment, developing strategies for reclaiming ownership of one's body, and finding inspiration through stories of empowerment, individuals can achieve greater emotional and physical well-being. These practices foster a deeper connection between the mind and body, promoting holistic healing and a sense of empowerment.

CHAPTER 9. Navigating Emotional Flashbacks
9.1 Understanding Emotional Flashbacks
9.2 Identifying Triggers
9.3 Techniques to Manage Flashbacks
9.4 Long-Term Strategies for Coping

Emotional flashbacks are intense and often debilitating experiences for individuals with complex PTSD (C-PTSD) and other trauma-related disorders. Unlike visual flashbacks that involve reliving a traumatic event, emotional flashbacks are sudden and overwhelming surges of emotional states, such as fear, shame, or despair, that can transport a person back to the feelings they experienced during past trauma. This chapter will delve into understanding emotional flashbacks, identifying triggers, managing flashbacks, and developing long-term coping strategies.

9.1 Understanding Emotional Flashbacks

Definition and Characteristics: Emotional flashbacks are characterized by the sudden onset of intense emotional distress that can be overwhelming and disorienting. They often involve regressive feelings of being small, helpless, and powerless, similar to what was experienced during the original trauma. According to Pete Walker, author of "Complex PTSD: From Surviving to Thriving," emotional flashbacks can "catapult a person instantly into a state of emotional and physical regression"

Symptoms: Symptoms of emotional flashbacks include anxiety, panic, feelings of worthlessness, deep-seated shame, and despair. Individuals may also experience physical symptoms such as rapid heartbeat, sweating, and trembling. These symptoms can last from a few minutes to several hours, making daily functioning challenging.

Impact on Daily Life: Emotional flashbacks can severely impact a person's daily life, affecting their ability to work, maintain relationships, and engage in regular activities. The unpredictability and intensity of these flashbacks can lead to avoidance behaviors, social isolation, and increased anxiety about potential triggers.

9.2 Identifying Triggers

Identifying triggers is a crucial step in managing emotional flashbacks. Triggers can be specific situations, people, places, sounds, smells, or even internal states that evoke memories or feelings associated with past trauma.

Common Triggers:
Common triggers for emotional flashbacks include:

- Interpersonal Conflicts:
Arguments or confrontations can remind individuals of past abuse or neglect.

- Authority Figures:
Encounters with authority figures can trigger feelings of powerlessness and fear.

- Sensory Cues: Specific smells, sounds, or visual stimuli that were present during the original trauma can act as triggers.

- Emotional States:

Feelings of vulnerability, shame, or fear can trigger a flashback, as these emotions are closely tied to the trauma experience.

Self-Reflection and Journaling:
Keeping a journal can help individuals track their emotional flashbacks and identify patterns and triggers. Noting the circumstances and emotional states preceding a flashback can provide valuable insights.

Therapeutic Techniques:
Therapists often use techniques such as guided self-reflection and trauma narratives to help clients identify and understand their triggers. Cognitive-behavioral therapy (CBT) and other trauma-focused therapies can be particularly effective in this process.

Case Study: Maria:
 Maria, a 35-year-old woman, experienced frequent emotional flashbacks triggered by interactions with her boss, who reminded her of a controlling parent. Through journaling and therapy, Maria identified the similarities between her boss's behavior and her parent's abuse. This awareness helped her develop strategies to manage her emotional responses in these situations.

9.3 Techniques to Manage Flashbacks

Managing emotional flashbacks involves a combination of immediate coping strategies and long-term therapeutic approaches. The following techniques can help individuals regain control during a flashback and reduce its intensity.

Grounding Techniques:
Grounding techniques help individuals anchor themselves in the present moment, reducing the intensity of the flashback. Examples include:

- 5-4-3-2-1 Technique:
Identify five things you can see, four things you can touch, three things you can hear, two things you can smell, and one thing you can taste.

- Deep Breathing:
 Practice deep, slow breathing to calm the nervous system. Focus on inhaling deeply through the nose and exhaling slowly through the mouth.

- Physical Grounding:
Engage in physical activities such as walking, stretching, or holding a grounding object like a smooth stone.

Self-Compassion:
Practicing self-compassion involves treating oneself with kindness and understanding during a flashback. Dr. Kristin Neff emphasizes, "Self-compassion involves being warm and understanding toward ourselves when we suffer, fail, or feel inadequate, rather than ignoring our pain or flagellating ourselves with self-criticism"

Mindfulness and Meditation:
Mindfulness and meditation practices can help individuals stay present and observe their thoughts and emotions without judgment. Regular practice can increase emotional regulation and reduce the frequency and intensity of flashbacks.

Safe Place Visualization:
Visualizing a safe and calming place can provide comfort and security during a flashback. This technique involves imagining a location where the individual feels safe, peaceful, and protected.

Therapeutic Support:
Working with a therapist who specializes in trauma can provide essential support and guidance. Therapists can teach coping strategies, offer validation, and help process the underlying trauma contributing to the flashbacks.

Case Study:
John: John, a 40-year-old military veteran, struggled with emotional flashbacks related to combat experiences. His therapist introduced him to grounding techniques and mindfulness practices. John found that practicing deep breathing and visualizing a safe place helped him manage his flashbacks more effectively. With continued therapy, John's flashbacks became less frequent and intense.

9.4 Long-Term Strategies for Coping

Developing long-term strategies for coping with emotional flashbacks involves building resilience, enhancing self-awareness, and integrating therapeutic practices into daily life.

Building Resilience:
Building resilience involves strengthening the ability to adapt and recover from adversity. This can be achieved through:
- Healthy Lifestyle Choices:
Regular exercise, a balanced diet, and sufficient sleep can improve overall well-being and resilience.
- Social Support:
Building a supportive network of friends, family, and community can provide a buffer against stress and enhance resilience.
- Stress Management:
 Learning and practicing stress management techniques, such as relaxation exercises and time management, can reduce overall stress levels.

Enhancing Self-Awareness: Increasing self-awareness involves understanding one's emotional and physical responses to stress and trauma. This can be achieved through:
- Regular Self-Reflection: Regularly reflecting on one's thoughts, feelings, and behaviors can increase self-awareness and identify patterns that contribute to flashbacks.
- Therapeutic Practices: Engaging in therapeutic practices such as journaling, art therapy, or talking with a therapist can enhance self-awareness and facilitate healing.

Integrating Therapeutic Practices:

Integrating therapeutic practices into daily life can provide ongoing support and reduce the impact of flashbacks. This includes:

- Routine Grounding Exercises:
Incorporating grounding exercises into daily routines can help maintain emotional stability and reduce the frequency of flashbacks.
- Mindfulness and Meditation:

Regular mindfulness and meditation practice can enhance emotional regulation and increase present-moment awareness.

- Ongoing Therapy:
Continuing therapy, even after symptoms improve, can provide ongoing support and prevent relapse.

Case Study:
Sarah: Sarah, a 30-year-old woman with a history of childhood trauma, developed a comprehensive coping plan with her therapist. This plan included regular exercise, mindfulness meditation, and maintaining a strong support network. Sarah also continued therapy to process unresolved trauma. Over time, Sarah built resilience, increased self-awareness, and developed effective strategies for managing emotional flashbacks.

Quotations from Experts

- Pete Walker: "Emotional flashbacks are sudden and often prolonged regressions into the intense, overwhelming feeling-states of childhood abuse and neglect. They are the child's feelings of overwhelming fear, shame, alienation, rage, grief, and depression."

- Dr. Kristin Neff: "Self-compassion involves being warm and understanding toward ourselves when we suffer, fail, or feel inadequate, rather than ignoring our pain or flagellating ourselves with self-criticism."

Academic and Book References

The understanding and management of emotional flashbacks are well-documented in academic literature and therapeutic practice. Key references include:

- "Complex PTSD: From Surviving to Thriving" by Pete Walker: This book provides a comprehensive guide to understanding and managing complex PTSD, including techniques for navigating emotional flashbacks.
- "The Body Keeps the Score" by Dr. Bessel van der Kolk: This book explores the impact of trauma on the body and mind, emphasizing the importance of addressing emotional flashbacks in trauma therapy.
- "Self-Compassion: The Proven Power of Being Kind to Yourself" by Dr. Kristin Neff: This book offers insights into the practice of self-compassion and its benefits for individuals with trauma-related disorders.

Conclusion

Navigating emotional flashbacks requires a multifaceted approach that includes understanding the nature of flashbacks, identifying triggers, employing immediate coping techniques, and developing long-term strategies for resilience and self-awareness. By integrating therapeutic practices into daily life and seeking ongoing support, individuals can manage and reduce the impact of emotional flashbacks, leading to improved emotional and physical well-being.

CHAPTER 10. Integration and Moving Forward

10.1 Integrating Somatic Practices
10.2 Daily Life Applications
10.3 Strategies for Long-Term Healing
10.4 Maintaining Progress Beyond Therapy

Integrating somatic practices into daily life and moving forward after trauma is essential for achieving sustained healing and well-being. This chapter explores how to incorporate somatic techniques into everyday routines, strategies for long-term healing, and maintaining progress beyond therapy. By understanding and applying these principles, individuals can continue their journey towards holistic recovery.

10.1 Integrating Somatic Practices

Integrating somatic practices involves incorporating body-based techniques into regular routines to support ongoing healing. Somatic practices emphasize the connection between the mind and body, helping individuals process and release trauma stored in their bodies.

Core Concepts:
Somatic therapy focuses on bodily sensations, movements, and the body's role in processing emotions and trauma. Dr. Peter Levine, a pioneer in somatic therapy, explains, "Trauma is not what happens to us, but what we hold inside in the absence of an empathetic witness"
[[1](https://lifearchitect.com/integrating-somatic-techniques-in-therapy/)].

Mindful Awareness:
Developing mindful awareness of the body's sensations is a foundational aspect of somatic practices. This involves paying

attention to physical sensations, movements, and breath without judgment. Regular mindfulness meditation can enhance this awareness and help individuals stay present.

Daily Routines:
Integrating somatic practices into daily routines can provide consistent support for healing. This includes incorporating activities such as yoga, tai chi, and breathwork into morning or evening routines. Dr. Bessel van der Kolk emphasizes the importance of these practices: "The most important issue for traumatized people is to find a sense of safety in their own bodies"

Case Study: Emma:
Emma, a 35-year-old woman recovering from childhood trauma, found that integrating somatic practices into her daily routine significantly improved her well-being. She started her day with a 10-minute mindfulness meditation, practiced yoga three times a week, and used breathwork exercises during stressful moments. These practices helped Emma develop a stronger connection to her body and reduced her anxiety and emotional distress.

10.2 Daily Life Applications

Applying somatic practices in daily life involves incorporating techniques that promote body awareness and emotional regulation into everyday activities. These applications can enhance overall well-being and support long-term healing.

Mindful Movement:
Engaging in mindful movement practices such as yoga, tai chi, or qigong can promote physical and emotional balance. These practices combine movement, breathwork, and mindfulness, helping individuals stay grounded and present.

Breathwork: Breathwork techniques can be used throughout the day to manage stress and regulate emotions. Practices such as diaphragmatic breathing, box breathing, and alternate nostril breathing can be easily incorporated into daily routines.

Body Scans:
Regular body scans can help individuals become more aware of physical sensations and areas of tension. This practice involves mentally scanning the body from head to toe, noticing any sensations without judgment. Body scans can be done at any time, such as during a break at work or before bed.

Grounding Exercises:
Grounding exercises help individuals anchor themselves in the present moment, reducing the intensity of distressing thoughts and emotions. Techniques such as the 5-4-3-2-1 exercise, deep breathing, and physical grounding (e.g., feeling the ground beneath your feet) can be practiced regularly.

Case Study: David:
 David, a 40-year-old man with a history of trauma, incorporated somatic practices into his daily life to manage his symptoms. He practiced mindful movement through tai chi every morning, used breathwork techniques during stressful situations, and did a body scan before bed each night. These practices helped David stay grounded, reduce his anxiety, and improve his overall well-being.

10.3 Strategies for Long-Term Healing

Long-term healing involves developing strategies that promote sustained recovery and prevent relapse. These strategies focus on building resilience, maintaining a support network, and continuing therapeutic practices.

Building Resilience:
Resilience is the ability to adapt and recover from adversity.
Building resilience involves:
- Healthy Lifestyle Choices:
Engaging in regular exercise, eating a balanced diet, and getting sufficient sleep can improve overall well-being and resilience.

- Social Support:
Building a supportive network of friends, family, and community can provide a buffer against stress and enhance resilience. Dr. Gabor Mate emphasizes the importance of social support: "The nature of trauma is that it disconnects us from our bodies, from our feelings, and from our relationships. Healing involves reconnecting to those aspects of ourselves and our lives" - Stress Management: Learning and practicing stress management techniques, such as relaxation exercises, time management, and mindfulness, can reduce overall stress levels.

Maintaining Therapeutic Practices: Continuing therapeutic practices beyond formal therapy can support long-term healing. This includes:

- Routine Grounding Exercises:
 Incorporating grounding exercises into daily routines can help maintain emotional stability and reduce the frequency of distressing symptoms.

- Mindfulness and Meditation:
 Regular mindfulness and meditation practice can enhance emotional regulation and increase present-moment awareness.

- Ongoing Therapy:

Continuing therapy, even after symptoms improve, can provide ongoing support and prevent relapse. Regular check-ins with a therapist can help address any emerging issues and maintain progress.

Case Study: Sarah:
Sarah, a 30-year-old woman with complex PTSD, developed a comprehensive coping plan with her therapist. This plan included regular exercise, mindfulness meditation, and maintaining a strong support network. Sarah also continued therapy to process unresolved trauma. Over time, Sarah built resilience, increased self-awareness, and developed effective strategies for long-term healing.

10.4 Maintaining Progress Beyond Therapy

Maintaining progress beyond therapy involves integrating therapeutic practices into daily life and seeking ongoing support. This includes continuing to practice self-care, staying connected with a support network, and remaining vigilant for signs of relapse.

Self-Care Practices: Engaging in regular self-care practices can help individuals nurture and honor their bodies. This includes activities such as taking relaxing baths, practicing skincare routines, and engaging in activities that bring joy and relaxation.

Continued Learning and Growth:
Continuing to learn about trauma and healing can empower individuals and provide new insights and techniques for managing symptoms. Reading books, attending workshops, and participating in support groups can provide valuable resources for ongoing healing.

Support Network:
Staying connected with a support network is essential for maintaining progress. This includes maintaining relationships with friends, family, and community members who provide emotional support and encouragement.

Case Study: Mike:
Mike, a veteran with PTSD, successfully integrated somatic practices into his daily life. He continued to practice yoga, meditation, and breathwork after completing therapy. Mike also joined a support group for veterans, which provided a sense of community and ongoing support. By maintaining these practices and staying connected with his support network, Mike was able to sustain his progress and manage his symptoms effectively.

Quotations from Experts

- Dr. Peter Levine: "Trauma is not what happens to us, but what we hold inside in the absence of an empathetic witness."
- Dr. Bessel van der Kolk: "The most important issue for traumatized people is to find a sense of safety in their own bodies."
- Dr. Gabor Mate: "The nature of trauma is that it disconnects us from our bodies, from our feelings, and from our relationships. Healing involves reconnecting to those aspects of ourselves and our lives."

Academic and Book References

The importance of integrating somatic practices and moving forward after trauma is well-documented in academic literature and therapeutic practice. Key references include:

- "The Body Keeps the Score" by Dr. Bessel van der Kolk: This book explores the impact of trauma on the body and mind, emphasizing the importance of integrating somatic practices for healing.
- "Waking the Tiger: Healing Trauma" by Dr. Peter Levine: This book introduces the principles of Somatic Experiencing and provides practical techniques for integrating somatic practices into daily life.
- "When the Body Says No: The Cost of Hidden Stress" by Dr. Gabor Mate: This book explores the connection between stress, trauma, and physical health, highlighting the importance of integrating mind-body practices for long-term healing.

Conclusion

Integrating somatic practices into daily life and moving forward after trauma involves developing mindful awareness, incorporating body-based techniques into regular routines, and building resilience. By maintaining therapeutic practices, staying connected with a support network, and continuing to learn and grow, individuals can achieve sustained healing and well-being. These practices foster a deeper connection between the mind and body, promoting holistic recovery and a sense of empowerment.

CHAPTER 11. Support Systems and Community Healing
11.1 Importance of Support Networks
11.2 Building a Supportive Community
11.3 Role of Group Therapy
11.4 Community Healing Initiatives

Support systems and community healing play a critical role in the recovery journey for individuals who have experienced trauma. This chapter explores the importance of support networks, strategies for building a supportive community, the role of group therapy, and various community healing initiatives. These elements collectively contribute to a holistic healing process that extends beyond individual therapy.

11.1 Importance of Support Networks

Support networks, comprising family, friends, and community members, provide essential emotional and practical support for trauma survivors. These networks offer a sense of belonging, validation, and empathy, which are crucial for recovery.

Emotional Support:
Emotional support from loved ones helps trauma survivors feel understood and less isolated. It provides a safe space to express feelings and experiences without judgment. Dr. Judith Herman, a renowned trauma expert, emphasizes, "Recovery can take place only within the context of relationships; it cannot occur in isolation"

Practical Support: Practical support includes assistance with daily tasks, financial help, and navigating healthcare systems. This type of support can alleviate stress and allow survivors to focus on their healing journey.

Case Study: Sarah:
Sarah, a 30-year-old woman recovering from sexual assault, found immense support in her friends and family. They provided emotional support by listening to her experiences and offering comfort. Additionally, they helped her with daily tasks and accompanied her to therapy sessions, making her feel less alone and more supported in her recovery journey.

11.2 Building a Supportive Community

Building a supportive community involves creating connections and fostering an environment where individuals feel safe, accepted, and valued. This process can significantly enhance the healing journey for trauma survivors.

Creating Safe Spaces: Establishing safe spaces, both physical and emotional, where individuals can share their experiences and feelings without fear of judgment or retribution is crucial. These spaces can be formal, such as support groups, or informal, like gatherings with friends and family.

Encouraging Open Communication: Open and honest communication within a community fosters trust and mutual support. Encouraging individuals to share their stories and listen to others can create a sense of solidarity and understanding.

Community Programs and Activities: Engaging in community programs and activities that promote well-being and social connection can enhance the sense of belonging and support. Examples include community yoga classes, art therapy workshops, and group outings.

Case Study: Mike:

Mike, a veteran with PTSD, struggled with isolation and anxiety after returning from service. He joined a local veterans' group that provided a safe space to share his experiences. The group also organized community activities like hiking and meditation sessions, which helped Mike build connections and feel supported in his healing process.

11.3 Role of Group Therapy

Group therapy is a powerful therapeutic approach that leverages the healing potential of communal support. It provides a structured environment where individuals can share their experiences, learn from others, and receive feedback and encouragement.

Benefits of Group Therapy:
- Shared Experiences: Group therapy allows individuals to connect with others who have similar experiences, reducing feelings of isolation and validating their emotions.
- Mutual Support: Members of the group provide emotional support to each other, fostering a sense of community and shared healing.
- Skill Building: Group therapy sessions often include activities and discussions that build coping skills, emotional regulation, and interpersonal communication.

Therapeutic Techniques:
Various therapeutic techniques can be used in group therapy, including cognitive-behavioral therapy (CBT), dialectical behavior therapy (DBT), and psychodynamic therapy. These techniques help address the diverse needs of group members.

Case Study: Jane:
Jane, a survivor of childhood abuse, participated in a trauma-focused group therapy program. The group provided a safe

space for her to share her story and receive support from others with similar experiences. Through the group's CBT sessions, Jane learned effective coping strategies and gained a sense of empowerment and resilience.

11.4 Community Healing Initiatives

Community healing initiatives aim to address trauma at both individual and collective levels. These initiatives often involve collaborative efforts from various stakeholders, including healthcare providers, community organizations, and local governments.

Public Awareness Campaigns:
Raising awareness about trauma and its impact through public campaigns can reduce stigma and encourage individuals to seek help. These campaigns can also promote understanding and empathy within the broader community.

Support Groups and Workshops:
 Organizing support groups and workshops focused on trauma recovery can provide valuable resources and support for individuals. These groups offer a safe space for sharing experiences, learning coping strategies, and building community connections.

Integrative Health Programs:
Integrative health programs that combine traditional and alternative therapies can address the holistic needs of trauma survivors. These programs may include yoga, meditation, art therapy, and other body-based practices.

Policy Advocacy:
Advocating for policies that support trauma-informed care and mental health services is crucial for long-term community

healing. This includes promoting access to mental health resources, funding for trauma recovery programs, and training for healthcare providers.

Case Study: Community Healing Project:
 A community healing project in a small town aimed to address the collective trauma experienced after a natural disaster. The project involved public awareness campaigns, support groups, and integrative health programs. Through these efforts, the community members were able to come together, share their experiences, and support each other in the healing process. The project also advocated for better mental health services and trauma-informed care in local healthcare facilities.

Quotations from Experts

- Dr. Judith Herman: "Recovery can take place only within the context of relationships; it cannot occur in isolation."
- Dr. Bessel van der Kolk: "Trauma affects the entire community, and recovery must involve the entire community. Healing is a collaborative and communal process."

Academic and Book References

The importance of support systems and community healing is well-documented in academic literature and therapeutic practice. Key references include:

- "Trauma and Recovery" by Dr. Judith Herman: This book explores the stages of trauma recovery and emphasizes the importance of relationships and community in the healing process.
- "The Body Keeps the Score" by Dr. Bessel van der Kolk: This book delves into the impact of trauma on the body and mind, highlighting the role of community and collective healing.

- "Group Therapy for Trauma: A Practical Guide" by Dr. Judith Lewis Herman: This guide provides practical insights and techniques for conducting group therapy for trauma survivors.

Conclusion

Support systems and community healing are integral to the recovery process for trauma survivors. By understanding the importance of support networks, building a supportive community, utilizing group therapy, and engaging in community healing initiatives, individuals can achieve holistic healing and resilience. These elements foster a sense of belonging, validation, and empowerment, contributing to long-term well-being and recovery.

CHAPTER 12. Case Studies and Personal Stories
12.1 Real-Life Examples of Somatic Healing
12.2 Personal Narratives of Recovery
12.3 Lessons Learned from Survivors
12.4 Inspirational Journeys of Transformation

Exploring real-life examples and personal stories of somatic healing provides profound insights into the transformative power of this therapeutic approach. This chapter delves into various case studies, personal narratives, lessons learned, and inspirational journeys, highlighting the resilience and strength of trauma survivors.

12.1 Real-Life Examples of Somatic Healing

Case Study: Emma's Journey with Somatic Experiencing
Emma, a 28-year-old woman, experienced chronic anxiety and panic attacks following a traumatic car accident. Traditional talk therapy provided some relief, but her symptoms persisted. Emma's therapist recommended somatic experiencing, a body-oriented approach developed by Dr. Peter Levine. Through somatic experiencing, Emma learned to focus on her bodily sensations and gradually release the trauma stored in her body. Over several months, her panic attacks decreased significantly, and she regained a sense of control and calmness. Emma's case illustrates the efficacy of somatic experiencing in addressing trauma's physical and emotional components.

Case Study: John's Recovery through Trauma-Sensitive Yoga
John, a 45-year-old military veteran, struggled with PTSD and emotional numbness after returning from combat. He found it challenging to engage in traditional therapy due to his heightened arousal state and avoidance behaviors. His therapist introduced him to trauma-sensitive yoga, which

combines gentle yoga practices with a focus on safety and body awareness. Through consistent practice, John reconnected with his body, learned to manage his arousal levels, and experienced a reduction in PTSD symptoms. John's story underscores the value of incorporating body-based practices in trauma therapy, particularly for those with intense physical and emotional responses.

Case Study: Maria's Healing with EMDR and Somatic Techniques

Maria, a survivor of childhood sexual abuse, faced debilitating flashbacks and dissociation. Her therapist used Eye Movement Desensitization and Reprocessing (EMDR) alongside somatic techniques to help Maria process her traumatic memories. By integrating EMDR's focus on eye movements and somatic awareness of bodily sensations, Maria could reprocess her memories and release the trauma stored in her body. Over time, her flashbacks diminished, and she felt more grounded and present. Maria's case highlights the synergistic effects of combining EMDR with somatic therapies for comprehensive trauma treatment.

12.2 Personal Narratives of Recovery

Personal Narrative: Sarah's Story of Resilience
Sarah, a 30-year-old woman, faced multiple traumas throughout her life, including domestic violence and a severe illness. She struggled with depression, anxiety, and a negative body image. Sarah found solace in a support group that emphasized body positivity and healing through movement. She began attending dance therapy sessions, which allowed her to express her emotions and reconnect with her body in a safe, supportive environment. Over time, Sarah developed a stronger sense of self-worth and resilience. Her narrative

demonstrates the power of community and movement in fostering healing and recovery.

Personal Narrative: David's Journey to Self-Acceptance
David, a 40-year-old man, experienced childhood neglect and emotional abuse. He carried deep-seated shame and self-loathing into adulthood, impacting his relationships and career. David sought help through a somatic therapy program that combined mindfulness, bodywork, and self-compassion exercises. As he progressed in therapy, David learned to identify and challenge his negative self-beliefs, gradually developing self-acceptance and compassion. His journey to self-acceptance was transformative, allowing him to build healthier relationships and pursue his passions. David's story highlights the profound impact of somatic therapies on self-perception and emotional healing.

Personal Narrative: Emily's Transformation through Breathwork
Emily, a survivor of sexual assault, experienced chronic tension and difficulty breathing. She felt disconnected from her body and often experienced panic attacks. Emily's therapist introduced her to somatic breathwork, a practice that focuses on conscious breathing to release tension and trauma. Through regular breathwork sessions, Emily learned to regulate her breathing, release physical tension, and reconnect with her body. Her panic attacks became less frequent, and she developed a sense of inner peace and empowerment. Emily's transformation through breathwork illustrates the importance of addressing the body's needs in trauma recovery.

12.3 Lessons Learned from Survivors

Survivors of trauma offer valuable lessons about resilience, healing, and the importance of a holistic approach to therapy.

These lessons can inspire and guide others on their healing journeys.

Lesson 1: The Body Remembers

One of the most critical lessons from trauma survivors is that the body holds onto traumatic experiences. Dr. Bessel van der Kolk, author of "The Body Keeps the Score," emphasizes, "Trauma is stored in the body, and the body needs to be part of the healing process" [[1](https://www.besselvanderkolk.com/resources/the-body-keeps-the-score)]. Survivors have shown that addressing the physical manifestations of trauma is essential for comprehensive recovery.

Lesson 2: Healing is Non-Linear

Recovery from trauma is not a straightforward path. Survivors often experience setbacks and progress in a non-linear fashion. Understanding and accepting this can help individuals maintain patience and compassion for themselves. Sarah's narrative of resilience highlights the importance of recognizing and celebrating small victories on the healing journey.

Lesson 3: The Power of Community

Survivors consistently emphasize the importance of community and support networks in their recovery. Whether through support groups, therapy, or informal connections, having a supportive community can provide validation, empathy, and encouragement. David's journey to self-acceptance was significantly influenced by the support and understanding he received from his therapy group.

Lesson 4: Integrating Multiple Therapies
Combining different therapeutic approaches can enhance the healing process. Survivors like Maria have benefited from integrating therapies such as EMDR and somatic techniques,

which address both cognitive and physical aspects of trauma. This holistic approach can provide more comprehensive and effective treatment.

Lesson 5: Self-Compassion is Key

Developing self-compassion is a crucial component of healing. Survivors like David have found that learning to be kind and understanding towards oneself can significantly improve emotional well-being and foster resilience. Dr. Kristin Neff, a leading researcher in self-compassion, states, "Self-compassion involves being warm and understanding toward ourselves when we suffer, fail, or feel inadequate" [[2](https://www.self-compassion.org)].

12.4 Inspirational Journeys of Transformation

Inspirational Journey: Mike's Path to Empowerment

Mike, a veteran with PTSD, struggled with feelings of helplessness and anger. Through a combination of somatic experiencing, mindfulness meditation, and group therapy, Mike began to regain a sense of control over his life. He learned to manage his symptoms, reconnect with his body, and develop a more positive outlook. Mike's journey to empowerment inspired many in his community, showing that healing and transformation are possible even after severe trauma.

Inspirational Journey: Jane's Triumph over Trauma

Jane, a survivor of childhood abuse, faced years of depression and self-doubt. She found healing through a trauma-focused yoga program that emphasized body awareness and emotional expression. Jane's commitment to her practice allowed her to release the trauma stored in her body and develop a sense of inner strength. She eventually became a yoga instructor, using her story to inspire and help others on their healing journeys.

Jane's triumph over trauma demonstrates the transformative power of body-based therapies.

Inspirational Journey: Emily's Advocacy and Activism
After recovering from sexual assault, Emily channeled her healing into advocacy and activism. She used her experiences to raise awareness about sexual violence and promote somatic therapies as a path to recovery. Emily founded a non-profit organization that provides resources and support for survivors, helping them access holistic healing practices. Her journey from survivor to advocate highlights the potential for personal transformation to create broader social change.

Quotations from Experts

- Dr. Bessel van der Kolk: "Trauma is stored in the body, and the body needs to be part of the healing process."
- Dr. Peter Levine: "Trauma is not what happens to us, but what we hold inside in the absence of an empathetic witness."
- Dr. Kristin Neff: "Self-compassion involves being warm and understanding toward ourselves when we suffer, fail, or feel inadequate."

Academic and Book References

The transformative power of somatic healing is well-documented in academic literature and therapeutic practice. Key references include:

- "The Body Keeps the Score" by Dr. Bessel van der Kolk: This book explores the impact of trauma on the body and mind, highlighting the importance of integrating somatic practices for comprehensive healing.
- "Waking the Tiger: Healing Trauma" by Dr. Peter Levine: This book introduces the principles of Somatic Experiencing and

provides practical techniques for addressing trauma through the body.
- "Self-Compassion: The Proven Power of Being Kind to Yourself" by Dr. Kristin Neff: This book offers insights into the practice of self-compassion and its benefits for trauma survivors.

Conclusion

Real-life examples, personal narratives, and inspirational journeys underscore the profound impact of somatic healing on trauma recovery. By integrating body-based practices, fostering self-compassion, and building supportive communities, individuals can transform their lives and achieve holistic healing. These stories of resilience and transformation provide hope and guidance for others on their healing journeys, demonstrating that recovery is possible and empowering.

CHAPTER 13
Weekly Plan of Exercises and Activities for Healing the Wounds of a Raped Woman

Healing from sexual trauma is a multifaceted process that involves physical, emotional, and psychological recovery. Here is a weekly plan of exercises and activities designed to support a woman's healing journey. This plan incorporates elements of somatic therapy, mindfulness, and community support.

Day 1: Mindfulness and Grounding
Morning:
- Mindful Breathing Exercise: Spend 10 minutes practicing deep, mindful breathing. Focus on the breath as it enters and leaves the body, allowing the mind to become calm and centered.
- Grounding Exercise: Engage in the 5-4-3-2-1 grounding technique to connect with the present moment. Identify five things you can see, four things you can touch, three things you can hear, two things you can smell, and one thing you can taste.

Afternoon:
- Gentle Yoga: Attend a trauma-sensitive yoga class or follow an online session that emphasizes gentle movements and body awareness.

Evening:
- Journaling: Write about your thoughts and feelings. Reflect on the day's experiences and any emotions that arose during mindfulness and yoga.

Day 2: Physical Activity and Support
Morning:

- Walking: Take a 20-minute walk in a peaceful environment. Focus on the sensation of your feet touching the ground and the rhythm of your steps.

Afternoon:
- Support Group: Attend a support group meeting for survivors of sexual trauma. Sharing experiences and hearing from others can provide comfort and validation.

Evening:
- Relaxation: Practice progressive muscle relaxation for 15 minutes. Tense and then relax each muscle group, starting from your toes and moving up to your head.

Day 3: Breathwork and Self-Compassion
Morning:
- Breathwork Session: Engage in a 10-minute breathwork exercise. Focus on deep, diaphragmatic breathing to release tension and promote relaxation.

Afternoon:
- Art Therapy: Spend an hour creating art. Use drawing, painting, or any other medium to express your emotions and experiences.

Evening:
- Self-Compassion Meditation: Practice a 15-minute self-compassion meditation. Repeat phrases like, "May I be kind to myself," and "May I find peace and healing."

Day 4: Body Awareness and Movement
Morning:
- Body Scan Meditation: Perform a 15-minute body scan meditation to increase awareness of physical sensations and areas of tension.

Afternoon:
- Dance Therapy: Participate in a dance therapy session or simply dance to your favorite music at home. Allow your body to move freely and expressively.

Evening:
- Reading: Read a chapter from a book on healing from trauma, such as "The Body Keeps the Score" by Dr. Bessel van der Kolk.

Day 5: Nature and Connection
Morning:
- Nature Walk: Spend 30 minutes walking in nature. Pay attention to the sights, sounds, and smells around you. Allow nature to soothe and ground you.

Afternoon:
- Connecting with a Friend: Meet with a trusted friend for coffee or a meal. Share your thoughts and feelings in a supportive environment.

Evening:
- Guided Imagery: Engage in a 15-minute guided imagery exercise. Imagine a safe and peaceful place where you feel completely secure and relaxed.

Day 6: Creative Expression and Reflection
Morning:
- Creative Writing: Spend 30 minutes writing creatively. This could be poetry, a short story, or a personal essay that reflects your journey.

Afternoon:

- Therapy Session: Attend a therapy session with a trauma-informed therapist. Discuss your progress and any challenges you are facing.

Evening:
- Gratitude Journal: Write down three things you are grateful for today. Reflect on positive experiences and moments of joy.

Day 7: Rest and Renewal
Morning:
- Meditation: Practice a 20-minute meditation focusing on relaxation and inner peace.

Afternoon:
- Massage or Bodywork: Schedule a massage or bodywork session to release physical tension and promote relaxation.

Evening:
- Reflection and Planning: Reflect on the past week and plan for the upcoming week. Identify any adjustments needed to support your healing journey.

THE END